Keto Diet Food List

What to Eat and Avoid on The Keto Diet

By: Bring On Fitness

Bring On Fitness

© Copyright 2018 – Bring On Fitness – All Rights Reserved.

The contents of this book may not be reproduced, duplicated, or transmitted without direct written permission from the author.

Under no circumstances will any legal responsibility or blame be held against the publisher for any reparation, damages, or monetary loss due to the information herein, either directly or indirectly.

Legal Notice:

This book is copyright protected. This is only for personal use. You cannot amend, distribute, sell, use, quote, or paraphrase any part or the content of this book without the consent of the author.

Disclaimer Notice:

Please note the information contained in this document is for educational and entertainment purposes only. Every attempt has been made to provide accurate, up-to-date, complete, and reliable information. No warranties of any kind are expressed or implied. Readers acknowledge that the author is not engaging in the rendering of legal, financial, medical, or professional advice. The content of this book has been derived from various sources. Please consult a licensed professional before attempting any techniques outlined in this book.

By reading this document, the reader agrees that under no circumstances is the author responsible for any losses, direct or indirect, which are incurred as a result of the use of

Bring On Fitness

information contained within this document, including, but not limited to, errors, omissions, or inaccuracies.

About Bring On Fitness

Our passion for fitness gave life to **Bring On Fitness**. We started with the goal of helping as many people as we can. To educate, motivate and to help change peoples lives for the better. Bring On Fitness is not only for the fitness enthusiasts, but also for the beginner. We strongly believe nothing is more important than learning the basics and creating a strong foundation in both nutrition - through meal planning, and in exercise - by following a specific plan. This is just as important for the beginner, as it is for the experienced athlete.

We set high standards for ourselves, the information we share, and the products we carry. Our goal is to provide you with exceptional products that suit your needs and the knowledge and motivation to help you work towards and achieve your health and fitness goals.

Keep up to date by liking us on Facebook and Instagram @bringonfitness

And for a complete list of reads and a FREE GIFT check us out at: www.bringonfitness.com

"Our Mission is to have a positive impact in changing peoples lives. We will deliver the best possible fitness and nutrition solutions that will empower people to achieve their health and fitness goals."

Bring On Fitness

Table Of Contents

Introduction 11

Chapter One: An introduction to the Ketogenic Diet 13

   How does the ketogenic diet affect metabolism? 13

      Ketosis versus Calorie Restriction *14*

      Metabolic Benefits of Ketosis *15*

      Ketosis and Insulin *16*

   Exercise and the ketogenic diet 16

   The benefits of the ketogenic diet 16

      Reduced appetite *16*

      Weight loss *17*

   Better Mental Focus 17

      More Energy *18*

      Fights Type II Diabetes *18*

      Increases levels of HDL Cholesterol *19*

      Low Blood Pressure *19*

Chapter Two: How to Shift into the State of Ketosis 21

   Step 1: Reduce your intake of carbohydrates 21

Step 2: Increase Physical Activity 22

Step 3: Increase the intake of healthy fats 23

Step 4: Maintain Adequate Protein Intake 23

Step 5: Your body now produces ketones 24

Chapter Three: Food to Eat and Avoid 27

Food to Eat 27

Eggs 27

Olive oil and olives 28

Meat, Seafood, and Poultry 28

High-fat Dairy 29

Dark Chocolate 29

Berries 30

Cruciferous Vegetables 30

Avocado 31

Coconut oil 31

Food to Avoid 32

Starches and Grains 32

Alcohol 32

Sugar 33

Conclusion 35

About Bring On Fitness 37

Bring On Fitness

Introduction

Thank you for purchasing the book, "Keto Diet Food List: What to Eat and Avoid on The Keto Diet."

Most people have stopped caring about their health. They are often so worried about their finances or other aspects of their lives that they forget about their food and lifestyle. Obesity has become a common health disorder today, and it is only now that people have started to understand the consequences of obesity.

It is important to maintain your weight because it has a mental, physical, and psychological impact on your body. There are different exercise routines, diet regimens, and diet supplements that are available to you. However, how do you know which of these options is good for your body and which is not? Your goal must be to choose the option that is healthy for you.

You shouldn't just change what you eat, but you must also change the way you think. You must choose a course of action that will help you reach your ideal weight. This is where the ketogenic diet comes in. Through this diet, you can change your lifestyle and also embrace a low-carb diet that will change your life.

Many people are unaware of what the ketogenic diet is. This book provides you with information on what the ketogenic diet is and how it changes your metabolism. When you are on the ketogenic diet, your body shifts into a metabolic state called ketosis. In this metabolic state, your liver burns fatty acids to

Bring On Fitness

produce ketones, which are used by some parts of the body as a source of energy. This book also lists the different types of food you are allowed to eat and what to avoid when you follow the ketogenic diet.

Thank you once again for purchasing this book. I hope you gather all the information you need.

Chapter One: An introduction to the Ketogenic Diet

The ketogenic diet is a low-carb and high-fat diet that transforms your body into a fat-burning machine through the process of ketosis. This diet is referred to by many different names – low-carb diet, low-carb high-fat diet, etc. There are many proven benefits of this diet, which are discussed in the later part of this chapter.

When you eat food that is high in carbohydrates, your body produces glucose and insulin. The former is a molecule that the body converts into energy. It is easier for the body to break glucose down into energy molecules; therefore, it will choose to attack glucose molecules before it looks for other energy sources. Insulin is produced by your body to break glucose molecules down into the bloodstream and transport those molecules around the body. As glucose is used as the primary source of energy, the fat in your body is not needed and is, therefore, stored.

How does the ketogenic diet affect metabolism?

This section gives you an overview of metabolism and ketosis.

If you follow a normal or a high-carbohydrate diet, your body will only use glucose as the main source of energy. When you reduce your carbohydrate intake, your body will enter into a metabolic state called ketosis. Your body will begin to target the fat in your body and break that fat down into ketone bodies that can be used as energy sources by some parts of the body.

Let us look at how ketosis can be used to maintain a healthy metabolism.

Ketosis versus Calorie Restriction

It is not effective to lose weight simply by reducing your caloric intake. Many doctors and scientists have conducted research to understand this concept better. They have identified that a decrease in your caloric intake alone can harm your metabolism and also lower your metabolic rate. If you want to understand this better, look at the winners of the show Biggest Loser. When the contestants reduced their caloric intake, their metabolism dropped, which led to weight loss for a few months, followed by weight gain.

Research has shown that the body reacts differently when you fast. The metabolic response of your body to fasting is different and healthy.

- An increase in growth hormones, which results in the maintenance of lean muscle mass.
- A steep drop in insulin, which prevents the resistance of the body to insulin.
- An increase in the norepinephrine hormone, which helps to keep basal metabolism high.

When the glycogen from carbohydrates is fully used, the body begins to burn through the fat reserves, which is a basic survival mechanism of the human body.

Metabolic Benefits of Ketosis

The body shifts into the metabolic state of ketosis when you fast. When you follow the ketogenic diet, you push your body into a state of nutritional ketosis, which is the process of burning the fatty acids in the body while eating a good quantity of protein and healthy fats. When you push your body into the state of nutritional ketosis through the ketogenic diet, you will reap the benefits of going into ketosis and fasting without causing any harm to your metabolism.

When the body turns to its fat stores for fuel, metabolism is maintained because the body is producing energy. However, if you reduce your caloric intake, you will slow down your metabolism. Additionally, when your body learns to burn fatty acids instead of glucose to produce energy, you will reap multiple benefits, including:

- Less inflammation
- A higher percentage of fat being burned
- Better immunity
- Increased longevity
- Better mental clarity
- Protection of the brain
- Prevention and protection against cancer

Ketosis and Insulin

People often develop multiple problems associated with metabolism when their body stops responding to insulin. When your body becomes resistant to insulin, there will be a higher concentration of glucose in your bloodstream, which can lead to type II diabetes and other disorders. Research has concluded that a carbohydrate-restricted diet controls insulin levels when the body is fasting.

Exercise and the ketogenic diet

The effects of the ketogenic diet are profound and visible when you exercise. When you start the ketogenic diet, it will be difficult to perform exercise because your body is learning to switch from glucose to fat reserves to produce energy. Start with at least 20 minutes of exercise when you begin the ketogenic diet, and gradually increase the time you spend on exercise.

The benefits of the ketogenic diet

Reduced appetite

Most people tend to consume more food when they are on a diet because they are unable to control their cravings. When you reduce your intake of carbohydrates, your body starts to burn fatty acids to produce energy. When your body learns to use fatty acids to produce energy, it will not require too much glucose, which helps to reduce your cravings. Multiple studies have been conducted to understand how a low-carb diet is different from and better than a low-fat, high-carb diet. These studies have concluded that the former helps to reduce the appetite.

Weight loss

Most people follow a diet to lose weight. When you follow the ketogenic diet, the fat reserves become the primary source of energy. How does this happen?

When your body enters the metabolic state called ketosis, the insulin and blood sugar levels drop, which gives the fat cells the ability to release any water they may have been retaining. It is for this reason that most people see a drop in their weight. Once the water has been released, the fat cells reduce in size and find it easy to navigate through the bloodstream and reach the liver, where they are converted into ketones. This process will continue as you progress and reduce your intake of carbohydrates.

Better Mental Focus

The issue with carbohydrates being used as a source of energy is that they cause a fluctuation in your blood sugar levels that causes an inconsistency in the amount of energy produced. This inconsistency makes it hard for your brain to stay focused for a long time. When your body is in the state of ketosis, your brain uses ketones to produce energy. As this source of energy is consistent, your brain can focus for a long time, which leads

Bring On Fitness

to an active mind. It is a hard feeling to explain because you never realize that your mind is not functioning at its best when you eat too many carbohydrates. When you follow the ketogenic diet, you can observe these changes in a day or two.

More Energy

There is a limit to the amount of glycogen that can be stored by the body, which means that you must constantly eat to maintain your energy levels. However, there is plenty of stored fat that your body can work with, and your body can store more fat, which means that your body can never run out of fuel, as it has a renewable source of fuel. Therefore, you are always energetic throughout the day. Have you ever wished for a day when you do not need to take a nap after lunch? Well, that is the lifestyle of a person who follows a ketogenic diet.

Fights Type II Diabetes

People who have type II diabetes have increased production of insulin in their bloodstream. Given that the ketogenic diet reduces the intake of carbohydrates, the body reduces the production of insulin, thereby reversing type II diabetes. Multiple studies have concluded that the ketogenic diet helps to control the key symptoms that lead to type II diabetes.

Increases levels of HDL Cholesterol

People often panic when they read the above statement, but there are two types of cholesterol – LDL and HDL. The latter is the good cholesterol that moves the cholesterol in the body into the liver where it is either excreted or reused. The former carries cholesterol to other parts of the body other than the liver. When you follow the ketogenic diet, the HDL cholesterol levels increase in the body, thereby reducing the risk of heart disease.

Low Blood Pressure

High blood pressure is an indicator of heart problems, and the ketogenic diet helps to maintain blood pressure. There are times when people suffering from high blood pressure have stopped taking their medicine when they integrated the ketogenic diet into their lives.

Bring On Fitness

Chapter Two: How to Shift into the State of Ketosis

The previous chapter gave you an overview of what ketosis is and how it is beneficial to the human body. That being said, it takes planning and work to achieve the state of ketosis. Your body does not shift into the state of ketosis if you simply reduce your intake of carbohydrates. You must put in some extra effort to ensure that your body is constantly in the state of ketosis to reap the benefits of the ketogenic diet. This chapter covers some steps that can be followed to shift your body into the state of ketosis.

Step 1: Reduce your intake of carbohydrates

It is important to consume a low-carb diet to achieve the state of ketosis. Your body often uses glucose as the main source of energy. However, different cells in your body can use other sources of fuel. These sources include ketones and fatty acids. Your body stores glucose in your muscles and liver in the form of glycogen. When you reduce your carbohydrate intake, the glycogen stored by the body is reduced, which allows the release of fatty acids in your body. Your liver converts these acids into ketone bodies, such as beta-Hydroxybutyrate, acetone, and acetoacetate, which are used by different parts of the brain as fuel.

Bring On Fitness

The amount of carbs that an individual is allowed to consume depends on that individual alone. Some people may need to limit their carbohydrate intake to 20 grams a day, whereas there are others who can consume twice that amount of carbohydrates and still shift to the state of ketosis. These limits are only advised for people who want to control blood sugar levels, lose weight, and reduce the risk of heart diseases.

A therapeutic ketogenic diet that is used to treat epilepsy or used as an experimental treatment for cancer is to limit the intake of carbohydrates to 15 grams per day to increase ketone levels.

Step 2: Increase Physical Activity

Many studies have shown that ketosis helps to improve the performance of some athletes. Additionally, being active can help you move into the state of ketosis with ease. When you exercise, glycogen stores are used to provide your body with fuel. These stores are replenished when you consume a diet that is high in carbohydrates, which are broken down into glucose and then converted to glycogen. However, when you reduce the intake of carbohydrates, the glycogen stores are not fully replenished, and in response, the liver increases the production of ketones that are used as the source of fuel for the muscles.

A study concluded that when exercise is performed at low blood ketone levels, the rate at which ketones are produced increases. However, when the blood ketone levels are already high, the level does not increase but may decrease when exercise is performed. It is true that your body produces more

Keto Diet Food List

ketones when you exercise, but it may take your body at least four weeks to use fatty acids and ketones as sources of fuel.

Step 3: Increase the intake of healthy fats

When you consume healthy fats, your bloodstream ketone levels increase. This helps to shift your body into the state of ketosis. It is important to remember that the ketogenic diet is low in carbohydrates but is high in fat. However, a high intake of fat does not translate into increased ketone levels in the bloodstream.

A study conducted for three weeks had 11 healthy people as subjects and compared the effects of the different fat intakes with the effects of fasting on ketone levels in the body. The ketone levels were similar in people who consumed either 80% or 90% of their caloric intake from fat.

As it is important to consume more fat on a ketogenic diet, it is important that you choose high-quality sources. The following chapter lists some of the best sources of fat that you must consume when you are on the ketogenic diet. However, if your goal is to lose weight, you must ensure that you do not consume too many calories in total.

Step 4: Maintain Adequate Protein Intake

If you wish to achieve ketosis fast, you have to ensure that your protein intake is not excessive but just the right amount. The ketogenic diet designed to treat epileptic patients restricts the consumption of both carbohydrates and protein to increase ketone levels. Studies are being conducted to understand whether this diet can be beneficial for cancer patients because it is believed that this version of the ketogenic diet helps to limit tumor growth. However, it is not healthy to cut back on proteins to increase the production of ketones in your body.

It is important to consume the right amount of protein to provide the liver with enough supply of amino acids that can be used to make new glucose for the parts of the body that do not use ketones or fatty acids to produce energy. The protein intake should also be high enough to repair tissue and maintain muscle mass, especially when the carbohydrate intake is low. Weight loss often results in the loss of both fat and muscle; therefore, it is essential that you consume the required amount of protein to ensure that you do not lose too much muscle.

To calculate the ideal intake of protein for your body on a ketogenic diet, multiply your body weight by 0.55 to 0.77. For example, if your body weight is 120 pounds, your intake should be 66 – 92.4 grams.

Step 5: Your body now produces ketones

Given that your carbohydrate intake has decreased, there is limited glucose available for the body to use as fuel. Your body begins to attack the fat reserves and use the fatty acids available to produce energy. The fatty acids enter the bloodstream and move to the liver, where they are broken down to form ketone bodies. Use an appliance that will help you identify whether your body is in the state of ketosis. You will start to lose weight when your body is shifted into the state of ketosis.

Bring On Fitness

Chapter Three: Food to Eat and Avoid

This chapter covers the list of foods that you should eat and those that you should avoid.

Food to Eat

Eggs

Eggs are considered one of the most versatile and healthiest foods. Many experts suggest that eggs are a type of "superfood."

The thirteen essential minerals and vitamins and the antioxidants that protect the eye, such as zeaxanthin and lutein, are found in eggs. The yolk is also the best source of choline, which is a methyl donor and an essential nutrient that is involved in multiple physiological processes.

Egg yolks do contain high levels of cholesterol, but the consumption of yolks does not affect the blood cholesterol levels in many people. Some studies have concluded that eggs can modify the shape of the LDL cholesterol to reduce the risk of any heart disease. The consumption of eggs keeps the levels of blood sugar stable and also gives a feeling of satiation. Therefore, this leads to a decrease in caloric intake, which means that eggs are a superfood that aids weight loss.

Bring On Fitness

One large egg only contains one gram of carbs and close to 6 grams of protein. This makes it the perfect keto-friendly health food.

Olive oil and olives

Olives and virgin olive oil contain many health-promoting compounds and oleocanthal, which is a phenolic compound and is one of those that ae studied the most. This compound has anti-inflammatory properties that are similar to that of ibuprofen, which makes use of olive oil and olives. This is a great addition for those who want to reduce inflammation and pain.

Meat, Seafood, and Poultry

You may have heard about how poultry, seafood, and meat are food groups that are rich in protein. However, did you know that these food groups contain certain essential vitamins and minerals that are not found in plant food? Vitamin B12 is an essential nutrient because it is a highly absorbable form of creatine, iron, carnosine, DHA, and taurine that is found in abundance in animal products. Poultry and fresh meat are packed with several minerals, along with Vitamin B. It is best to have 100% grass-fed meat and pasture-raised poultry to ensure that you obtain the required levels of nutrients. These products contain more antioxidants than grain-fed meat products. The same can be said about shellfish; however, it is important to understand the number of carbohydrates present in different types of fish. Most people following the ketogenic diet often consume more protein because they like meat and seafood. However, it is important to spread the amount of protein consumed between meals to ensure that you do not lower your ketone levels.

High-fat Dairy

High-fat dairy contains high-quality protein, conjugated linoleic acid, vitamins, and minerals. A combination of these nutrients is necessary to maintain bodily functions and strength as you age. A recent study was conducted to understand the effect of high-fat dairy on aging people. The study concluded that the consumption of seven to ten ounces of ricotta cheese increased the muscle strength and mass of older participants. In simple words, always ask for extra cheese. You do not have to be cheap with cream, butter, and cheese when you follow the ketogenic diet. Given that high-fat dairy contains low carbohydrates, it is best to include a reasonable amount of any dairy product in every meal.

Dark Chocolate

This is a guilty pleasure that is good for your body. This chocolate contains flavonol that decreases the risk of heart disease, insulin resistance, and blood pressure. Cocoa is often called a "superfruit" because it contains the same number of antioxidants as any other keto-friendly fruit. This does not mean that you can consume as much dark chocolate as you can lay your hands on when you are on a ketogenic diet. Every chocolate contains a decent amount of net carbs that will kick your body out of ketosis. When you buy any cocoa product or chocolate, you must read the label and ensure that there are no added sugars. You should also look at the number of carbs per serving of the chocolate.

Berries

Most fruits are rich in carbohydrates and cannot be consumed on a ketogenic diet; however, some berries are exceptions. There are different types of berries, and each type contains different kinds of anthocyanins. These compounds are responsible for the color of the berries and also have anti-inflammatory effects on the body. For example, studies have concluded that wild blueberries prevent inflammation in the brain and improve memory as you age. When you follow the ketogenic diet, you must consume moderate amounts of berries because they have high net carbohydrate content.

Cruciferous Vegetables

Vegetables that are low in carbohydrates are rich in fiber, antioxidants, vitamins, and minerals, and cruciferous vegetables have an added health boost. These vegetables are rich not only in Vitamins A and K but also in sulforaphane. The latter is a compound that is created when you chew or crush cruciferous vegetables. When the compound is digested, it activates a protective shield around cells to prevent oxidation. It is for this reason that cruciferous vegetables decrease the risk of cancer and heart diseases and improve cognitive function. Cruciferous vegetables like kale and broccoli can be used as substitutes for foods that are rich in carbohydrates.

Avocado

Avocados must be consumed when you are on a ketogenic diet, especially when you have just started out because they are rich in several minerals and vitamins. Avocados are rich in potassium, and when you increase your potassium intake, you will be able to rid yourself of the keto flu during the initial days. Avocados are also known to improve triglyceride and cholesterol levels. If you are not a fan of avocados, you can use avocado oil instead. You may not get all the nutrients you need, but the oil contains monounsaturated fat, which helps improve the levels of cholesterol in the body.

Coconut oil

Coconut oil is known to help the body shift into the state of ketosis. This oil contains a fat called medium chain triglyceride (MCT), which is absorbed by the body and pushed into the liver, where it is converted into ketones or used to provide the body with energy. Coconut oil has four forms of MCTs; however, half of its fat comes from lauric acid. Studies show that fat sources that have a higher concentration of lauric acid produce higher levels of ketosis because this fat is broken down more slowly than other types of MCTs. MCTs can be used to induce the state of ketosis in children with epilepsy without reducing their intake of carbohydrates. When you add coconut oil to your diet, add it slowly to minimize any side effects like diarrhea and stomach cramps. Start with half a teaspoon per day and slowly work up to two teaspoons over the course of one week.

Food to Avoid

Starches and Grains

Most people consume bread in some form every day. It is convenient to run to the grocery store or Subway and pick up a sandwich. Bread is one food group that goes with every meal, and people avoid the ketogenic diet when they are asked to give up bread. Grains cause a lot of problems to the body. Recently, people have begun to switch to gluten-free food. When you cut grains out from your diet, you cut out tons of carbohydrates. You do not need to fret because people following the keto diet are innovative, and if they want to eat bread, they are going to find some way to do that. The same can be said for rice. If you want to consume rice, make yourself some cauliflower rice. Remember that where there is a will, there is a way in the keto world!

Alcohol

You must avoid alcohol regardless of which diet you follow. When you follow the ketogenic diet, you should watch your intake of carbohydrates and only worry about the drinks that are rich in carbohydrates. This means that you should give up on:

- Liqueurs
- Ciders
- Beer

You do not have to stay away from every type of liquor though, because most types of liquor are safe to drink when you follow a ketogenic diet. The following types of alcohol can be consumed when you follow a ketogenic diet:

- Gin
- Whiskey
- Scotch
- Tequila
- Vodka
- Rum
- Brandy
- Cognac

There are some types of alcohol that most drink straight up, but others do require something to be added. If you ever find yourself in a situation where you may have to consume a drink or two that could knock you out of ketosis, avoid or limit your intake.

Sugar

Fruit and candy are two of the favorite dishes that most people consume. When you start the ketogenic diet, you may need to give up on them, and this may break your heart. You may wonder how you can curb your cravings, but that is where fat

Bring On Fitness

bombs come in. Fat bombs provide you with all the sweets you need while also helping you reach the required fat content. However, you should be careful with the number of fat bombs you consume because you could be throwing yourself into a vicious cycle. You should completely avoid:

- Ice cream
- Fruit juices
- Pastries
- Cookies
- Sodas

If you love fruit, choose those that fit into the categories mentioned above, but watch your consumption.

Conclusion

Most people start the ketogenic diet when they are sure they want to lose weight. What they do not know is that one can reap multiple benefits when on the ketogenic diet. Over the course of the book, you have been introduced to the ketogenic diet and its benefits. You have also learned how the diet affects your metabolism and your body.

When you are on the ketogenic diet, your body moves into the metabolic state called ketosis. There are different ways to push your body into the state of ketosis. This book provides you with the steps that you must follow to switch to ketosis with ease. You have also learned about the different types of food you can consume and those you must avoid.

I hope you have gathered all the information necessary and wish you luck on your journey.

Thank you, and remember to share how well these Keto Diet Food List work for you. You can do that by writing a review in your Amazon account under Your Orders.

Thank you,

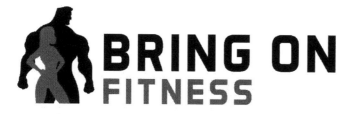

Bring On Fitness

About Bring On Fitness

Our passion for fitness gave life to **Bring On Fitness**. We started with the goal of helping as many people as we can. To educate, motivate and to help change peoples lives for the better. Bring On Fitness is not only for the fitness enthusiasts, but also for the beginner. We strongly believe nothing is more important than learning the basics and creating a strong foundation in both nutrition - through meal planning, and in exercise - by following a specific plan. This is just as important for the beginner, as it is for the experienced athlete.

We set high standards for ourselves, the information we share, and the products we carry. Our goal is to provide you with exceptional products that suit your needs and the knowledge and motivation to help you work towards and achieve your health and fitness goals.

Keep up to date by liking us on Facebook and Instagram @bringonfitness

And for a complete list of reads and a FREE GIFT check us out at: www.bringonfitness.com

"Our Mission is to have a positive impact in changing peoples lives. We will deliver the best possible fitness and nutrition solutions that will empower people to achieve their health and fitness goals."

Bring On Fitness

Made in the
USA
Middletown, DE